THE BIBLE CURE®

AND HEPATITIS C

DON COLBERT, M.D.

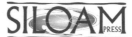

SILOAM PRESS

Living in Health—Body, Mind and Spirit

THE BIBLE CURE FOR HEPATITIS AND HEPATITIS C
by Don Colbert, M.D.
Published by Siloam Press
A part of Strang Communications Company
600 Rinehart Road
Lake Mary, Florida 32746
www.siloampress.com

Copyright © 2002 by Don Colbert, M.D.
All rights reserved

Library of Congress Catalog Card Number:
2002107571
International Standard Book Number: 0-88419-829-4

02 03 04 05 — 8 7 6 5 4 3 2 1
Printed in the United States of America

Wisdom From Above

If you have been diagnosed with hepatitis or hepatitis C, one of your greatest needs, though you may not realize it, is for God's wisdom. Learning to apply God's wisdom to your life can bring you the wonderful fruit of peace, happiness, rest and, ultimately, health. As you read through this Bible Cure booklet, you will discover how the wisdom of God can become a path to healing and health for you.

Equally important, God's wisdom will help you to live your life in a much better, happier and more peaceful way. We understand the power of divine wisdom from the Bible's beautiful description:

> The wisdom that comes from heaven is first of all pure; then peace-loving, con-siderate, submissive, full of mercy and

good fruit, impartial and sincere.

—JAMES 3:17, NIV

In these chapters we will explore ways in which God's wisdom can work for you as we take an in-depth look at hepatitis and hepatitis C. Prepare to discover how to apply His wisdom to your treatment regimen in a way that will allow God's healing power to touch your body, restore your good health and extend your life.

It is a startling fact that hepatitis and hepatitis C affect millions of Americans. If you or someone you love has been diagnosed with hepatitis or hepatitis C, even in the late stages of the disease, I want to encourage you with the fact that it is both treatable and beatable. And remember, God wants you well. To that end, He has provided wisdom and healing power to restore you to health.

In ancient civilizations, the liver was believed to be the seat of certain negative emotions. Scientifically, we understand that the liver's primary function is as a filter that rids the body of physical impurities. The ancients believed that the liver also "handled" the negative effects of emotional and spiritual impurities as well. They were convinced there was a vital connection between the liver's function and negative emotions such as anger, frustration and rage.

Interestingly, the prophet Jeremiah seems to support this notion when, during a time of intense emotional and spiritual turmoil, he cried out:

> Mine eyes do fail with tears, my bowels are troubled, my liver is poured out upon the earth, for the destruction of the daughter of my people; because the children and the sucklings swoon in the streets of the city
>
> —LAMENTATIONS 2:11, KJV

It is important to understand that your thinking patterns and emotional responses affect your body. God desires for you to be totally well, physically, mentally, emotionally and spiritually. As you discover the reality of the link between negative emotions and your liver's health, you will learn how to overcome the spiritual roots, as well as the physical cause, of liver disease.

An Exciting First Step

No matter what the root causes of your diagnosis for hepatitis or hepatitis C, by picking up this Bible Cure booklet you have taken an exciting first step toward renewed health. God's will is for your spiritual health as well as your physical health to be restored. He revealed His desire for you in the scriptures when the apostle John wrote:

> Dear friend, I am praying that all is well
> with you and that your *body* is as healthy
> as I know your *soul* is.
>
> —3 JOHN 2, EMPHASIS ADDED

With God's help, you can begin walking in physical and spiritual renewal. So as you begin to read through the pages of this booklet, get ready to win! This Bible Cure booklet is filled with hope and encouragement for understanding how to keep your body fit and healthy. In this book, you will

*uncover God's divine plan of health
for body, soul and spirit
through modern medicine, good nutrition
and the medicinal power
of Scripture and prayer.*

You will find key scripture passages throughout this book that will help you focus on the power of God. These divine promises will empower your prayers and redirect your thoughts to line up with God's plan of divine health for you—a plan that includes victory over hepatitis or hepatitis C and its destructive spiritual and physical roots.

In this Bible Cure booklet, you will gain a strategic plan for divine health in the following chapters:

1 Wisdom—a Pathway to Healing 1
2 Walking in Wisdom 18
3 Wisdom and Nutrition 37
4 Wisdom and Supplements 52
5 Wisdom and Healing
   Through Prayer 71

If you are suffering from hepatitis or hepatitis C, the chances are good that your body is experiencing a battle—and your mind and spirit as well. The truths in this booklet will arm you to win this intense conflict. With fresh confidence in the dynamic knowledge that God is real and that He loves you more than you could ever imagine, you can expect to enjoy complete restoration of your health.

It is my prayer that these powerful insights will bring health, wholeness and spiritual refreshing to you—body, mind and spirit. May they deepen your fellowship with God and strengthen your ability to worship and serve Him.

—DON COLBERT, M.D.

Chapter 1

Wisdom—a Pathway
to Healing

Wisdom is a pathway to life and health. The Bible clearly declares this reality:

> How blessed is the man who finds wisdom, and the man who gains understanding…Long life is in her right hand…She is a tree of life to those who take hold of her.
>
> —PROVERBS 3:13, 16, 18, NAS

> A wise man scales the city of the mighty, and brings down the stronghold in which they trust.
>
> —PROVERBS 21:22, NAS

Even if hepatitis or hepatitis C has become a "stronghold" in your body, the Bible assures you that wisdom will help to bring it down so that you

1

can reclaim your health and vitality. "Getting wisdom is the most important thing you can do!" declares the writer of Proverbs (Prov. 4:7). So, let's begin our conquering strategy of hepatitis and hepatitis C by gaining more understanding of their causes and symptoms, as well as the supplements needed to restore the liver. The wisdom gained will equip you to pull down this stronghold!

Brief Overview of the Liver

Next to your skin, your liver is your body's largest organ. It weighs about three pounds and is located just underneath the lower right rib cage.

Your liver has many duties. One of its most important functions is to purify or detoxify your body from the chemicals, toxins and other harmful substances you eat, drink and breathe in the environment in which you live. Everything that enters the bloodstream is presented to the liver's detoxification system eventually.

> *And the LORD will protect you from all sickness. He will not let you suffer from the terrible diseases you knew in Egypt, but he will bring them all on your enemies!*
> —DEUTERONOMY 7:15

One liter of blood every minute flows through

this giant filter where toxins are removed. The more toxins your liver eliminates from your body, the better you will feel. While the liver is filtering your blood and eliminating environmental as well as internal toxins, it is also performing many other important tasks, including:

- Processing all nutrients that come through the digestive tract
- Storing nutrients and releasing them when they are needed
- Maintaining hormonal balance
- Manufacturing bile, an important digestive juice
- Regulating cholesterol levels
- Cleaning waste products and bacteria from the blood
- Breaking down toxic substances, including medications, alcohol and drugs

We need the liver to function well to help convert the food we eat into energy. Its vital function of regulating cholesterol is also essential for forming sex hormones. In addition, your amazing liver creates vital enzymes, amino acids, hormones and proteins. Some of the proteins that your liver produces include:

- *Albumin,* which maintains fluid balance in the body
- *Clotting factors,* which are essential for the blood to clot
- *Enzymes,* which are involved in thousands of chemical reactions in the body

As you can see, any impairment to your liver can cause many different symptoms of disease.

Risks to a Healthy Liver

The world in which we live can be extremely dangerous to the health of the liver. More than one hundred drugs and medications in use today can harm the liver. Many very common chemicals and solvents with which we come in contact can also damage this vital organ. Some of the worst offenders are the chemicals used in dry cleaning.

Besides environmental and internal toxins, certain viruses are also known to inflame the liver, including hepatitis A, B and C viruses. These are the most common of the hepatitis viruses, though several others exist, including hepatitis D, E, F and G. Other viruses, such as the Epstein-Barr virus, the herpes simplex virus and the HIV virus can also inflame your liver.

Your liver can also be damaged by drinking too

much alcohol and by obesity. An abundance of toxins, use of drugs (including some medications), autoimmune liver disease and even some herbs can eventually inflame and damage your liver. But the most common cause of chronic hepatitis is the hepatitis C virus.

What Is Hepatitis C?

The word *hepatitis* means "inflammation of the liver." It comes from two Greek words: *hepato,* which means "liver," and *itis,* which means "inflammation." Hepatitis can be caused by anything that inflames or damages the liver; however, hepatitis C is caused by a virus.

Hepatitis C was discovered relatively recently and was first called the hepatitis C virus in 1989. Before this, it was simply known as non-A, non-B hepatitis. Testing for both hepatitis A and B was possible in the 1960s and 1970s. But blood tests to identify hepatitis C were not developed until 1990.

Hepatitis A is called "infectious hepatitis" because the virus spreads through contaminated food and water. This type of hepatitis is very common in Third World countries. Most of those who contract it recover their health. Victims of hepatitis A do not develop chronic infections.

Hepatitis B is a little different. It is called "serum hepatitis" because it is transmitted to others through blood and other body fluids. Most adults—95 percent—recover from hepatitis B, though a small percentage develops a chronic infection. Of the nearly 200,000 people who are infected by hepatitis B each year, only about 10,000 develop a chronic hepatitis B infection.

Hepatitis C is the most common chronic infection transmitted by the blood in the United States. However, unlike hepatitis B, of those

> *Jesus touched him. "I want to," he said. "Be healed!" And instantly the leprosy disappeared.*
> —MATTHEW 8:3

who contract hepatitis C, only 15 percent actually recover. Worldwide, nearly 150 million individuals suffer with chronic hepatitis C.

The Grim Facts

Hepatitis C is usually discovered when routine blood tests for life insurance or a physical exam indicate elevated liver enzymes. When this happens, a specific blood test for hepatitis C is usually administered. However, the routine blood test that includes liver function tests is not foolproof; about 30 to 50 percent of patients suffering with chronic hepatitis C have completely normal liver enzymes.

Approximately 10,000 Americans die each year from chronic hepatitis C. Projections show that mortality rates associated with hepatitis C will triple by the year 2015. According to the Centers for Disease Control, between 28,000 and 180,000 people are infected with hepatitis C each year. It is actually responsible for most liver transplants in the U.S. Once infected with the hepatitis C virus, about 20 percent of people go on to develop cirrhosis of the liver in about twenty years.

The Silent Epidemic

Hepatitis C is called the silent epidemic because so many people have the disease but are completely unaware of it. In fact, many times severe symptoms do not occur until the last stages of the disease—stages that may take decades to develop. What that means is a person can be walking around with advancing liver disease and never feel it or know it.

Since tests to screen the blood supply for the hepatitis C antibody were not developed until May 1990, it was impossible to know before then if donated blood contained hepatitis C or not. A more accurate blood test was available by May 1992, but by then many individuals had already received the virus through transfusions and organ transplants.

It is now believed that about one in fifty Americans has hepatitis C, and many are unaware that they are infected. The incidence

> *If you make the LORD your refuge, if you make the Most High your shelter, no evil will conquer you.*
> —PSALM 91:9–10

among African American males is thought to be the highest, with about one of every ten young African American men infected.

Hepatitis C is the most common cause of cirrhosis and liver cancer. *Baywatch's* Pamela Anderson's recent diagnosis with the disease has turned a national spotlight upon this silent killer.

A Closer Look at This Virus

The hepatitis C virus is a part of a family of viruses called the RNA viruses. These viruses invade liver cells in their attempt to make more viruses. The hepatitis C virus actually hijacks the cell and reprograms the cell's RNA and DNA, causing the liver cells to begin reproducing more viruses.

The millions of viruses formed in these liver cells eventually cause the cell to burst. An explosion of viruses is then released to infect other healthy cells. As the process continues, more and more liver cells are damaged, and many die.

Your body's immune system doesn't stand by idly as these viruses multiply. Your immune system instantly senses what is occurring and moves into action against this destructive process, working to neutralize the virus by making antibodies.

When this happens, the hepatitis virus recognizes the body's attempt to destroy it and turns into a chameleon to evade the immune system's defense. As an RNA virus, it is able to mutate or change its form. By doing so, it prevents the antibodies from attaching to it. While DNA viruses make billions of identical copies of themselves that antibodies can defend against, RNA viruses make billions of *similar,* not identical, viruses for which there is no defense.

Much of the damage that takes place in the liver as a result of these viruses invading it is caused by our own immune system. Simply put, our immune system attacks the virus but does not do it efficiently. So, the liver gets damaged in the process, similar to our military troops getting shot in "friendly fire" during war. This "friendly fire" damage to the liver is referred to as *immunopathic.*

The First Symptoms

When a person is first infected with hepatitis C, symptoms can range from very mild to quite severe. Usually, he develops flu-like symptoms with fever, chills, sweats, severe fatigue and nausea. Pain in the joints is not uncommon, as well as tenderness over the liver. It's even possible to develop diarrhea, a spastic colon and indigestion.

Hepatitis C may create psychological changes, such as mood swings, confusion, short-term memory loss, depression, restless sleep and irritability.

Some people with hepatitis C can no longer eat fatty foods or drink alcohol. Others may retain fluid in the legs and feet and experience abdominal bloating. Headaches and dizziness are not uncommon with acute hepatitis C infection.

Generally the flu-like symptoms subside along with the achy joints and muscles. But the chronic fatigue, irritable bowel and intolerance to fatty foods and alcohol tend to persist. A person with hepatitis C may also continue experiencing disturbed sleep, irritability and mood swings.

Advanced Stages

The progression of hepatitis C will continue for many years in the body, with or without major recognizable symptoms. Eventually, the effects of the virus will usually lead to more advanced stages of liver disease.

Chronic hepatitis C

As we have mentioned, 85 percent of people who have become infected with hepatitis C go on to develop chronic hepatitis. Only 15 percent of people overcome hepatitis C.

Cirrhosis of the liver

It usually takes a little more than twenty years for cirrhosis of the liver to develop.

Liver cancer

Approximately thirty years from the onset of hepatitis C, the virus may progress to liver cancer.

As the Disease Progresses

Most people with hepatitis C suffer relatively few symptoms. They may feel tired, experience insomnia and suffer with irritable bowel syndrome. However, the flu-like symptoms experienced at the onset of the disease only last a few weeks.

After those initial symptoms, for ten years or longer that same individual usually experiences few or no symptoms at all. But if hepatitis C is left untreated, the disease process can enter into the next stage of liver damage, which is called *fibrosis*.

Fibrosis is the scarring of the liver that results from the immune system fighting the infection for years. Eventually the liver begins to develop scar tissue where it has tried to repair the damage caused by the virus. When this happens, the liver is still able to function, but not at an optimal level.

> *News about him spread far beyond the borders of Galilee so that the sick were soon coming to be healed from as far away as Syria. And whatever their illness and pain, or if they were possessed by demons, or were epileptics, or were paralyzed—he healed them all.*
> —MATTHEW 4:24

That's why an individual with fibrosis will usually develop constant fatigue, irritable bowel syndrome and alcohol and fat intolerance.

The good news is that nearly two-thirds of all chronic hepatitis C sufferers will never progress beyond this stage. However, the remaining third of those with chronic hepatitis C will eventually progress to *cirrhosis* of the liver. Cirrhosis occurs when fibrosis becomes so severe that the structure and the function of the liver are seriously compromised.

In this state, blood can no longer flow freely through the liver. This can then lead to a state called *portal hypertension,* which is increased pressure in the portal vein caused by an obstruction of blood flow through the liver. This condition causes *ascites* to occur, which is severe abdominal swelling when the blood backs up in the portal vein and other abdominal veins and fluid is forced out of the veins and collects in the abdomen. Bleeding from esophageal varices (varicose veins of the esophagus) may also occur, along with *encephalopathy,* brain dysfunction caused from a liver unable to neutralize ammonia and causing confusion and memory loss.

Individuals with cirrhosis of the liver are at increased risk of developing *liver cancer.* About 20 percent of cirrhosis cases will advance to liver cancer. That's why an ounce of prevention is worth a pound of cure.

Treatable and Beatable

If you or a loved one has been diagnosed with hepatitis C, don't panic. Hepatitis C, especially if discovered early, is both treatable and beatable. Though it can be a very serious illness, even life threatening, that doesn't have to be the result for your life. There is much that you can do to help halt the progression of this disease even if you have some fibrosis of the liver. Because your immune system is critically important in the battle against this disease, learning to strengthen your immune system can help you win the battle.

So don't fear. With faith and godly wisdom, I believe that you can and will beat this disease. The Bible says, "Anything is possible if a person believes" (Mark 9:23).

As you continue to read, you will find a helpful outline of many powerful ways that you can combat and overcome hepatitis C in your body.

Conclusion

The very same healing power that was available during the time Jesus Christ walked the shores of Galilee raising the dead and seeing the lame jump up with joy is still available to you right now where you are. The Bible declares, "I am the Lord, and I do not change" (Mal. 3:6). God's healing power is as real today as it was when Jesus lived on earth.

That's not all. God's love and His desire to see you healed and whole hasn't changed either. No matter what stage of disease your body may be in, God can heal you. Reach out to Him today. Mix faith with wisdom as you learn to look to Him for your healing. He loves you more than you can ever know, and His love will not fail you.

As you get started in this Bible Cure, take a minute and let me pray with you for healing.

A BIBLE CURE PRAYER FOR YOU

Lord Jesus, thank You for dying on the cross to pay the price of salvation and wholeness—body, mind and spirit. I pray that Your precious Holy Spirit will visit this individual in a fresh and very special way as he or she reads this booklet. Let this one know in a deeper way than ever before that You are God, You are mighty, You are a healer, and Your healing power is available at this very minute. Cover Your precious child with a fresh blanket of wonderful love, and minister to all of his or her needs. In Jesus' wonderful name I pray. Amen.

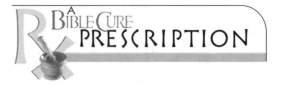

A BIBLE CURE PRESCRIPTION

Faith Builder

He was pierced through for our transgressions, He was crushed for our iniquities; the chastening of our well-being fell upon Him, and by His scourging we are healed.
—ISAIAH 53:5, NAS

Write out this verse and insert your own name into it: "He was pierced through for _____'s transgressions, He was crushed for _____'s iniquities; the chastening of _____'swell-being fell upon Him, and by His scourging _____ is healed."

Write out a personal prayer to Jesus Christ, thanking Him for exchanging His health for your pain. Thank Him for taking the power of sickness onto His own body so that He could purchase your healing from hepatitis or hepatitis C.

_____

_____

Chapter 2

Walking With Wisdom

Wisdom is a pathway that God has given us to walk upon. When we choose to walk in wisdom, the benefits to our lives and health are limitless. Walking on the path of godly wisdom will cause every day to get better, healthier, happier and brighter for us: "The path of the righteous is like the light of dawn, that shines brighter and brighter until the full day" (Prov. 4:18, NAS).

The benefits to walking on God's pathway of wisdom include health and healing. Scripture teaches us not to be wise in our own eyes. "Fear the Lord and turn away from evil. It will be healing to your body, and refreshment to your bones" (Prov. 3:7–8, NAS).

Each lifestyle choice that you and I make leads us down a pathway. Lifestyle choices can lead some down the pathway to hepatitis C.

Contracting Hepatitis C

You can only contract hepatitis C through contact with infected blood, which is why lifestyle choices are a key factor for many, though not all, in contracting hepatitis C. Mosquitoes and other insects do not transmit hepatitis C. Blood tainted with the hepatitis C virus must gain entry into the bloodstream through a cut or prick, or from blood splashing onto mucous membranes such as the eyes, nasal passages or the mouth. It can also gain entry into the bloodstream through the skin from an open sore. Therefore, exposure to other people's blood can cause a person to contract or spread this disease.

It will be helpful to discuss specific ways a person can be put at risk for contracting hepatitis C.

The risk of receiving blood transfusions

Receiving a blood transfusion cannot be considered a poor "lifestyle" choice; however, if you received a blood transfusion or organ transplant before 1990, it is important that you understand that you may have been exposed to tainted blood. Statistics show that one out of ten people who received a transfusion before 1990 contracted the hepatitis C virus.

Unfortunately, blood tests to detect the hepatitis C virus were not available before 1990. For that reason, those who had any surgery that required a blood transfusion before 1990 are at a significantly increased risk for the disease. Anyone who received hemodialysis prior to 1990 is at increased risk as well. A hemophiliac who received blood before 1990 has a much higher risk also.

The ELISA-1 test was developed in 1990 to detect hepatitis C. In 1992, the ELISA-2 blood test was developed, which is much more accurate than its predecessor. It would be wise for everyone who received a blood transfusion before 1990, and even before 1992, to be tested for the hepatitis C virus because of their increased risk.

The risk to IV drug users

Another way to contract hepatitis C is through IV drug use, especially from injecting drugs with dirty needles. Many people are infected with the hepatitis C virus because of a single use of injected drugs that happened twenty years prior.

It is important to know that hepatitis C is a much heartier virus than HIV, which is fragile. As a matter of fact, the hepatitis C virus can survive outside the body in microscopic traces of dried blood (on a needle, for example) for three months or even longer and still remain infectious.

The risk to cocaine users

Snorting cocaine is very irritating to the lining of the nose and often traumatizes the lining of the nostrils, causing nosebleeds. In fact, some of my patients who were formerly cocaine users actually have a hole in the nasal septum, which is the cartilage that separates the two nostrils.

Because the hepatitis C virus is hearty, it poses greater risk for infecting cocaine users. The nasal irritation caused by snorting cocaine can contaminate the straw or paper commonly used to snort cocaine with

> *As the sun went down that evening, people throughout the village brought sick family members to Jesus. No matter what their diseases were, the touch of his hand healed every one.*
> —LUKE 4:40

traces of dried blood. If the same straw or paper used by someone who has hepatitis C is used days, weeks or even months later by another person, the traces of dried blood left on the paper can still infect the user with the hepatitis C virus.

Interestingly, although written in ancient times, the Bible alludes to the evils of drug use when it

20

lists practices that keep us from entering the kingdom. Sorcery is listed along with immorality, impurity, sensuality and other evils of the flesh we are to avoid. (See Galatians 5:20.)

The Greek word translated "sorcery" is *pharmakeia,* from which we derive our word *pharmacy.* However, to the culture of the day it referred to producing a spell-giving potion by a "poisoner" or magician. God's Word declares that we must not use drugs in this wicked way. Obeying God's Word keeps us on a path of wisdom and good health.

The risk of tattoos and body piercing

Tattoos are becoming increasingly popular in today's culture. It used to be rare that anyone except members of the military or gang members would wear a tattoo. Now, however, basketball stars such as Allen Iverson and Dennis Rodman flamboyantly cover their bodies with tattoos.

Also, famous actors and actresses many times sport their own more modest tattoos. And tattoos are still very common among IV drug users, prostitutes, gang members and prisoners. Permanent eyeliner is also a type of tattooing, for which the same risk applies of contracting hepatitis C.

Getting a tattoo requires the use of a needle,

and that's where the problems arise. Before an individual is tattooed, his or her skin is shaved, and then ink is injected through the skin with a needle gun. If the needles, razor, ink or any other tattooing equipment used during the procedure are not sterile, then the hepatitis C virus can be transmitted to the person being tattooed.

It may surprise you to learn that even the ink can transmit the disease. Tattoo parlors are required by law to use sterile needles and new jars of ink for each new client. However, sterilization procedures vary. Some may be sloppy, and the ink may be reused. Remember, hepatitis C is a very hearty virus that can survive for months in traces of dried blood.

Body piercing is also enjoying increasing popularity in our culture. Today both young women and men not only get their ears pierced, but their navels, tongues and other body parts. If sterile needles are not used or if sterilization practices are sloppy, hepatitis C virus infection could occur. Even acupuncture needles that are reused and are not properly sterilized can place you at risk for hepatitis C infection.

Interestingly, the Bible forbids both tattooing and body piercing: "Ye shall not make any cuttings in your flesh for the dead, nor print any marks upon you: I am the LORD" (Lev. 19:28, KJV). The New American Standard Bible translates the passage this way: "You shall not make any cuts in your body for the dead, nor make any tattoo marks on yourselves: I am the LORD."

This was a commandment of God. Again, we see how choosing a lifestyle that pleases God and obeying His laws can protect our bodies from dangerous and life-threatening diseases.

Risk of multiple sex partners

Those who experience multiple sexual partners are also at a greatly increased risk of contracting hepatitis C. This especially applies to prostitutes and those have been with prostitutes. Because people who engage in this lifestyle are at a greatly increased risk of developing sexually transmitted diseases, many of which involve lesions or breaks in the skin or mucous membranes, such as herpes, it becomes easy for the hepatitis C virus to enter the body.

The Bible is very clear that God expects us to have sexual relations with our spouse only, and that should happen after we've been married. (See Exodus 20:14.) God's laws are not written to spoil our fun. As our loving Creator, He established rules and guidelines to protect us from harm because He cares for us. All of the destruction and death caused by sexually transmitted diseases we've experienced in our generation might have been avoided had we honored God's laws.

It is important to note that even if your spouse has hepatitis C, your risk of contracting the virus is very low. As a matter of fact, it's less than 5 percent. A few precautions that are advisable are to refrain from sexual intercourse during menstruation or use condoms to reduce the risk even further. And if you are the sexual partner of someone with hepatitis C, you should get tested.

> *He was wounded and crushed for our sins. He was beaten that we might have peace. He was whipped, and we were healed!*
> —Isaiah 53:5

Risk to healthcare workers

Unfortunately, even our heroes of today—doctors, nurses, firefighters, EMTs, police officers, lab technicians and so forth—run an increased risk of contracting hepatitis C through accidental needle pricks and from blood splashing on mucous membranes. Universal precautions to minimize such accidents are in place throughout the entire healthcare industry to help avoid this serious occupational hazard.

Others at risk

Because standards of cleanliness and sterilization procedures vary dramatically in medical facilities in Third World countries, anyone who has received invasive procedures or surgery in Third World countries should be considered at risk for hepatitis C.

Also, children born to women who are positive for hepatitis C are at risk for contracting the disease.

Finding a New Pathway

Even if we have broken God's laws and brought disease into our bodies, God still wants to see us well and healed. He is a loving Father who always wants what is best for us. He is not the condemning judge that religion has sometimes made Him to be.

The Bible declares His great love to us: "For God so loved the world that he gave his only Son that everyone who believes in him will not perish but have eternal life. God did not send his Son into the world to condemn it, but to save it" (John 3:16).

If lifestyle choices have brought disease into your body, don't condemn yourself; God does not condemn you. Ask God to forgive you for any bad choices and begin making better ones based upon godly wisdom. That's all repentance really is—a turning away from sin. Ask Jesus to come into your heart this very minute and He will. It's so simple!

He loves you so much. He's been waiting all of this time just to hear you ask Him to be your Savior and Healer. He is not just *a* healer; He is *your* healer. He gave His own life so that you

> *He personally carried away our sins in his own body on the cross so we can be dead to sin and live for what is right. You have been healed by his wounds!*
> —1 PETER 2:24

might be set free spiritually, mentally and physically. If you have never given your life to Jesus Christ and asked Him to come into your heart, I encourage you to take a minute and pray the prayer I have included at the end of this book. You'll be glad you did; He'll never disappoint you!

Who Should Get Tested?

Review the list below to see if you are among the individuals who have an increased risk of contracting hepatitis C and need to be tested.

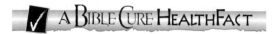

Are You at Risk?

- Anyone who received a blood transfusion or organ transplant before 1992
- Any hemophiliac or individual receiving hemodialysis prior to 1992
- Anyone who has injected drugs or shared needles
- Anyone who has snorted cocaine from a shared straw or piece of paper
- Anyone who has received a tattoo, body piercing or acupuncture treatment that could have involved improperly sterilized needles or ink that was reused
- Healthcare workers or anyone exposed to infected blood through needle pricks or from blood that came into contact with mucous membranes, such as the eyes, nose or mouth
- Anyone with multiple sexual partners, especially when involving prostitutes

HEALTHFACT HEALTHFACT HEALTHFACT HEALTHFACT HEALTHFACT HEALTHFACT HEALTHFACT

Don't let fear, embarrassment or denial keep you from getting tested. As you will see in the next chapters, there's much you can do to halt the progression of this disease and begin to see your body restored to vital health. Remember, also, that hepatitis C can lead to cirrhosis of the liver, which then places the person at increased risk of developing *liver cancer.* About 20 percent of cirrhosis cases will advance to liver cancer. That's why an ounce of prevention is worth a pound of cure.

Getting Tested

Here is some important information you will need to know as you or your loved one is tested for hepatitis C.

The most important test to diagnose hepatitis C is called the ELISA-II test, as we have mentioned. The ELISA-II test is able to detect hepatitis C antibodies. A second test, called the RIBA test (Recombinant Immunoblot Assay), is often used to confirm the diagnosis of hepatitis C.

Once it has been determined that a person has hepatitis C, it is important to have a viral load blood test to determine how much virus is present in the blood. The viral load is drawn before and during treatment of hepatitis C to determine how the patient is responding to treatment.

Hepatitis C is usually discovered when blood

tests show elevated liver enzymes. The most common enzyme elevated in hepatitis C is the SGPT or the ALT level. An elevated ALT level is usually a sign of inflammation of the liver. However, not all patients with hepatitis C have elevated ALT levels. In fact, approximately one-third of patients with hepatitis C have a normal ALT level. That is why it is so important to have the diagnostic test for hepatitis C (ELISA-II) if one has any other risk factors for hepatitis C.

A hepatitis C genotype test may also be performed to determine if one is more likely to respond to antiviral therapy. The genotype is the combination of genes within the hepatitis C virus, and there are six different genotypes. These six genotypes are subdivided into 1a, 1b, 2a, 2b and so on. Most patients with hepatitis C in the U.S. have genotype 1. Genotype 1a is the most common genotype, followed by 1b. Patients with genotype 1b tend to have less response to treatment and to have the disease progress more rapidly. The only way to determine the extent of damage to the liver by the hepatitis C virus is to have a liver biopsy. This is an outpatient procedure that has a very low complication rate. However, I recommend for best results that you choose a gastrointestinal specialist or a hepatologist who performs at least fifty or more liver biopsies a year.

Disease Stages

A liver biopsy will determine the stage of the disease. There are five main stages or categories that are actually based upon the degree of fibrosis or scarring that was seen in the liver biopsy:

- *Stage 0* means no inflammation or fibrosis. In other words, the liver appears normal.
- *Stage I* is liver inflammation only.
- *Stage II* is characterized with inflammation and early fibrosis in one part of the liver.
- *Stage III* is characterized by the liver having moderate to severe fibrosis throughout the liver.
- *Stage IV* is cirrhosis of the liver.

If you or a family member tests positive for hepatitis C, you will want to apply some wisdom to prevent family members from contracting it. Here are some tips for family members.

If a family member has hepatitis C, observe the following:

- Separate any sharp instruments including razors, clippers, manicure scissors or anything that could nick the skin to be used only by the family member with hepatitis C. Microscopic amounts of dried blood on an instrument are all it takes many times to infect a person with hepatitis C.
- Avoid sexual contact during menstruation, and dispose of sanitary napkins carefully.
- Do not share toothbrushes.

Note: Activities such as hugging and kissing do not transmit the virus unless there are sores or breaks in the skin around the lips or mouth. You also do not transmit the hepatitis C virus by sharing food or drinks.

Cautions for Hepatitis C Patients

If you have been diagnosed with hepatitis C, there

are some steps you should take to keep from causing your condition to worsen.

Avoid alcohol.

If you have hepatitis C, avoid drinking all alcoholic beverages. Alcohol puts the liver under stress and compromises the immune system, which needs to be strong to fight the hepatitis C virus. Alcohol also interferes with the liver's ability to regenerate and causes fat to build up in the liver (which can further compromise liver function), all of which usually leads to more rapid progression of hepatitis C to fibrosis and eventually cirrhosis.

Since your liver is already in a weakened state because of hepatitis C, drinking alcohol will compound the damage to your liver caused by hepatitis C. In fact, if you continue to drink excessively, you will be much more likely to develop cirrhosis of the liver and liver cancer.

Don't take drugs.

Most drugs exert some strain on the liver because the liver has to detoxify and break down most drugs and medications. Since your liver is already under attack, it's important to avoid medications and drugs unless they are absolutely necessary or unless they have been prescribed by a doctor who is aware of your condition. Particularly damaging to the liver is combining alcohol and Tylenol.

Shun environmental chemicals.

As we have mentioned, many environmental chemicals are also toxic to the liver and should be avoided. These include paints, solvents, petroleum-based chemicals, dry cleaning fluids and even chlorine.

A chemical that is particularly toxic to the liver is benzene, which is found in paints, paint thinners, many solvents, petroleum products, unleaded gasoline, pesticides and herbicides. It is important that you neither inhale the vapors of these chemicals nor allow them to contact the skin, since it can be absorbed into the skin.

Instead of drinking tap water, drink filtered water. In addition, attach shower filters to showerheads, which will help to filter out the chlorine.

Conclusion

When we make lifestyle choices according to God's wisdom, great promises become available to us. The Scriptures promise, "Watch the path of your feet, and all your ways will be established" (Prov. 4:26, NAS). Every godly choice you make is like a brick that helps pave a pathway for your life. Choice by choice you lay that pathway until your life arrives either at a safe place or a place of danger. So, build that pathway to health and life one step at a time. The choice is yours!

The Bible declares, "Today I am giving you a choice between prosperity and disaster, between life and death…Choose to love the Lord your God and to obey him and commit yourself to him, for he is your life" (Deut. 30:15, 20). I encourage you to choose the pathway of wisdom and discover new health, healing and a brand-new life in Jesus Christ.

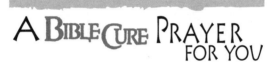

A BIBLE CURE PRAYER FOR YOU

Dear Jesus, I would like to know You better, to know the power of Your love and the peace of Your presence in my life. Teach me to walk in your pathway of wisdom that leads to wholeness and health. Thank You for dying on the cross to save and heal me. In Your mighty name, amen.

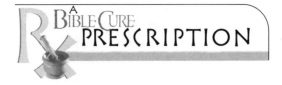

What behaviors have you been involved in that may have increased your risk of contracting hepatitis C?

_____

_____

What symptoms of hepatitis C have you experienced? (circle)

Fatigue

Irritable bowel syndrome

Insomnia

Intolerance to fatty foods

Irritability and mood swings

Others _____

What lifestyle changes will you make after reading this chapter?

_____

_____

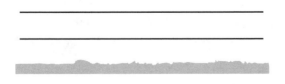

Chapter 3

Wisdom and Nutrition

There is healing power in wisdom: "The words of the wise bring healing" (Prov. 12:18); "The teaching of the wise is a fountain of life, to turn aside from the snares of death" (Prov. 13:14, NAS). God's wisdom applied to our dietary and nutritional choices is vital for those who are suffering from liver disease.

If you or a loved one has hepatitis C, what you eat will make a vast difference in your body's ability to heal. The nutrition you receive will protect and support your liver. A person who has hepatitis C but still has normal liver enzymes and a good appetite could eat almost anything without having symptoms; however, a patient with elevated liver enzymes or fibrosis commonly experiences irritable bowel syndrome, fat intolerance, diarrhea, indigestion and so forth.

In this chapter I will outline a dietary plan that would be wise for those individuals in all stages of hepatitis C; however, individuals with cirrhosis would also need special dietary instructions from their hepatologist or gastrointestinal specialist.

Lighten Your Liver's Load

The most important thing that you can do for your liver if you have chronic hepatitis C is to decrease its workload. Remember, the liver neutralizes and destroys toxins, metabolizes alcohol, cleanses the blood and removes waste products. It also processes all nutrients and stores carbohydrates, fats, proteins and vitamins.

It is vitally important for you to allow your liver to rest and recuperate. You can do this by avoiding foods that are especially demanding on the liver and eating foods that supply the liver and body with abundant nutrients. The following guidelines will help.

> *I will give you back your health and heal your wounds, says the LORD.*
> —JEREMIAH 30:17

Go organic.

Start eating only organic foods. Because they

are free from pesticides, metabolizing them will place less strain on the liver.

Eat free-range meats.

Choose free-range meats that do not contain the hormones, antibiotics and other chemicals that place additional stress on the liver.

Avoid fatty foods.

Foods that are high in fat place a strain on the liver since the liver must process those fats. Avoid or decrease your consumption of foods high in saturated fats found primarily in fatty cuts of meat, most dairy products and preserved meats.

Fried foods are especially hard on the liver and should be avoided. Avoid all hydrogenated or partially hydrogenated fats and refined oils. Instead of refined oils, choose modest amounts of extra-virgin or virgin olive oil.

Hydrogenated fats are found primarily in margarine and in most commercial brands of peanut butter, shortening and salad dressings. Partially hydrogenated fats are found in most baked goods, cookies, crackers, chips and most processed packaged foods.

Avoid all refined vegetable oils.

Corn oil, sunflower oil, safflower oil and almost

all vegetable oils found at supermarkets are generally high in lipid peroxides (free radicals). As such, they may be harmful to the liver.

Avoid peanuts.

Peanuts and peanut oil may contain traces of aflatoxin, a chemical that is formed by fungi and is very toxic to the liver. Therefore, avoid or decrease consumption of peanuts, peanut oil and peanut butter.

Avoid dairy products.

Intake of dairy foods should be reduced to a bare minimum. In their place, you should choose soy milk, rice milk or almond milk.

You may use modest amounts of clarified butter (called "ghee"), which has had all of the milk solids removed.

Avoid foods high in sugar.

Patients with hepatitis C also commonly have candida overgrowth in the small intestines. Sugar consumption aggravates this and weakens the immune system, our most powerful ally against hepatitis C. For more information on candida, refer to *The Bible Cure for Candida and Yeast Infections.* Viruses love sugar, so stop feeding the hepatitis C virus its favorite food—sugar.

Eat protein.

As we mentioned, your liver actually makes most of the proteins used by your body. Therefore, it's very important for you to eat sufficient amounts of different kinds of dietary protein in order to help your liver do its job.

Consume modest amounts of protein (3–4 ounces) for at least two meals of the day; also take a protein supplement such as whey or soy. Eat fish, chicken or turkey; white meat is preferred. Choose 3–4 ounces of extra-lean free-range beef in place of ground beef. However, red meat should not be consumed more often than once a week.

Individuals with hepatitis C usually have too much iron in the blood. Excessive iron can further harm the liver and feed the hepatitis C virus. Foods high in iron (such as beef liver, beef, iron-fortified cereals, bran, pumpkinseeds, blackstrap molasses, soynuts, spinach, red kidney beans, lima beans and prune juice) should be limited or avoided.[1]

> *He felt great pity for the crowds that came, because their problems were so great and they didn't know where to go for help. They were like sheep without a shepherd.*
> —MATTHEW 9:36

Avoid processed foods.

Drastically reduce your intake of processed foods because they usually contain many chemicals, including food additives and food colorings.

Avoid sugar substitutes.

Sugar substitutes such as NutraSweet and saccharin place an additional strain on the liver and should be avoided entirely. Instead, choose Stevia.

Decrease coffee and tea.

Decrease consumption of coffee and excessive amounts of tea, since caffeine also puts an additional strain on the liver. However, modest amounts of green teen (1 to 3 cups a day) are generally beneficial to the liver due to its powerful antioxidant effects.

Food Allergies

Many people with hepatitis C also have food allergies or sensitivities. It is important to find out what food allergies or sensitivities you may have and modify your diet accordingly. Common foods to which people have allergic reactions and sensitivities include eggs, dairy products and wheat.

An excellent test to determine food sensitivities is the Immuno One Bloodprint, a toxicity test by

ImmunoLabs. Your doctor can order this test by calling (800) 231-9197.

Eggs

Eggs may be eaten as a source of protein unless you are allergic to them. If you tolerate eggs, eating one whole egg along with two egg whites is a better choice than eating two or three whole eggs a day.

Dairy products

Dairy foods are the most common cause of food allergies. If you drink milk or eat dairy products, don't consume them on a daily basis. Whole milk is actually 4 percent milk with half of its calories coming from fat. When you drink 2 percent milk, you have reduced the fat calories to one-quarter coming from fat, which helps, of course. However, why not give your system a break and only use dairy products on occasion. Instead, try using almond milk, soy milk and even rice milk.

Wheat

Wheat contains gluten, which is a protein also found in oats, barley and rye; it is also a common food allergen. If you find that you are sensitive to wheat you need to avoid pasta, crackers, bagels, pretzels and all breads made with wheat, barley, oats and rye. You may substitute these allergy-causing foods with millet or brown rice bread.

Here is the check list of "no-no's" we have discussed that you should avoid to help restore health to your liver.

A BIBLE CURE HEALTH TIP

Foods to Avoid or Decrease Dramatically

- Alcohol
- Animal skins
- Excessive amounts of caffeinated beverages (modest amounts of green tea is OK)
- Dairy products (especially cheese, butter, ice cream, whole milk)
- Hydrogenated and partially hydrogenated fats
- Refined vegetable oils
- Fatty meats
- Simple sugars
- Peanuts and peanut butter
- Refined and processed foods
- Fried foods and fatty foods (especially saturated fats)
- Foods high in iron (such as liver, beef, iron-fortified cereals)
- Preserved meats (such as bologna, hot dogs, pepperoni)

Make Liver-Friendly Diet Choices

Liver maintenance is not difficult. You can promote the health of your liver by simply eating a liver-friendly diet. Make choices that include plenty of the following liver-friendly foods. They will help to cleanse and heal your liver.

Choose organic fruits.

Especially choose low-glycemic fruits, including Granny Smith apples, kiwis, blueberries, strawberries, blackberries and grapefruits. Fruit juice commonly causes diarrhea in patients with hepatitis C; therefore, I recommend consuming the fruit rather than drinking the juice.

Choose organic vegetables.

Eat as many raw vegetables as possible. When cooking fresh vegetables it's best to steam them instead of boiling them. Always remember that fresh vegetables contain more phytonutrients than canned or frozen vegetables. Preparing home-made vegetable soup is a delicious way to give your body a wide variety of vegetables. Use as many fresh, raw vegetables as possible, and try not to overcook them.

Cruciferous vegetables, including broccoli, cabbage, Brussels sprouts and cauliflower, are more important than others for liver detoxification. These liver-friendly vegetables contain potent phytonutrients such as indole-3-carbinol, sulforaphane and others, which aid the liver in detoxifying the body of chemicals and drugs. Of all the cruciferous vegetables, broccoli sprouts usually have the highest concentration of these phytonutrients. Here is a list of other liver-friendly vegetables that you should eat as often as you can:

- Artichokes
- Asparagus
- Beets
- Broccoli
- Brussels sprouts
- Cabbage
- Carrots
- Cauliflower
- Celery
- Chicory
- Garlic
- Leeks and onions
- Radishes

Choose liver-friendly starches.

Starches that the liver can tolerate better than others include brown rice, wild rice, rice pasta and brown rice bread. As we have mentioned, starches from wheat products, including breads, bagels, crackers, pasta, chips and cereals, should be limited or avoided altogether if you are sensitive to them or if you experience symptoms of diarrhea or irritable bowel syndrome after consuming them. Corn products may also need to be avoided by some individuals.

Choose liver-friendly fats.

The following fats are very good for your liver and for detoxification in general:

- Avocados
- Black currant seed oil
- Raw fresh nuts and seeds (avoid peanuts and cashews)
- Evening Primrose oil
- Borage oil
- Fish oil
- Flaxseed oil (but never cook with this oil)
- Extra-virgin olive oil

Beverages are important, too!

What you drink and how much you drink is just as important as what you eat. Here's a list of dos:

Juices. Juicing the vegetables listed on page 45 rather than fruits is very beneficial to the liver. For more information on juicing and some recipes, refer to my book *Toxic Relief.*

Teas. Green tea and other herbal teas (in moderation) make delicious beverages that will also promote liver health.

Water. Drink at least 2 quarts of filtered water a day.

Powerful detoxifying proteins

We have mentioned the importance of eating 3 to 4 ounces of good protein twice a day. One of the best sources of protein is from consuming fatty fish in your diet. Choose from the following list to add these powerful proteins to your diet for great detoxification.

- Salmon
- Halibut
- Herring
- Mackerel
- Free-range turkey (3–4 ounce serving)
- Free-range eggs
- Tuna (limit to one serving per week)
- Most other fish except for shellfish, catfish and swordfish
- Free-range chicken (3–4 ounce serving)

Having an occasional free-range egg will help supply the needed amino acids for Phase Two detoxification. I recommend combining one free-range egg with one or two additional free-range egg whites (eliminating the yolk). Also, please note the serving sizes and other cautions for the proteins listed above.

The Golden Rule of Liver Care

The most important rule of liver care can be simply stated: *Don't overeat.* Overeating places an enormous added burden on your liver and the detoxification pathways of your body. To assure liver health, only eat until you are satisfied and no more.

If you tend to be an overeater, here are some pointers that can help you change your eating patterns:

- In your home, serve individual plates of food with measured portions rather than having everyone serve themselves country style from bowls of food placed on the table. This will help to control portions and avoid the temptation to eat second servings just because the food is there.
- Eat more slowly. Chew each bite thirty times and place your fork on the table between bites. Give your brain a chance to tell your stomach how full it is getting before you decide to eat more.
- Plan a walk right after dinner rather than sitting and visiting at the dinner table where you may be tempted to overeat.

- When you eat at restaurants, try not to be a charter member of the "clean plate club." Restaurant portions are too large for most people to consume. Plan to take half of those enormous portions home in a doggy bag for the next day, or choose to split an entrée with your companion.

Conclusion

Even if a lack of wisdom in your life helped to cause liver disease, employing the sound wisdom of the nutritional guidelines we have discussed can help to turn your situation around.

Ask God to help you employ His wisdom with every bite of food you eat. As you do, you will begin to discover that wisdom truly is a fountain of life that delivers from the snares of death and disease. (See Proverbs 13:14.)

A BIBLE CURE PRAYER
FOR YOU

Dear Lord, teach me Your wisdom as I choose to take in foods that will help my body, especially my liver. Give me a spirit of self-control as I reach for various foods to satisfy and nourish my body. Thank You that You've provided Your wisdom for me to help me cleanse and support my body as it heals. Most of all, I thank You that You are the Divine Healer, and all healing comes from You. I ask You in Jesus' name to touch my body with Your healing power and repair the damage that hepatitis C may have caused. Free my body from this virus, and strengthen my immune system by Your supernatural power. In Jesus' name, I thank You. Amen.

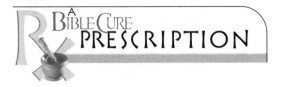

BIBLE CURE PRESCRIPTION

List the dietary changes you will begin making immediately to help strengthen and cleanse your liver.

_____

_____

List any foods or other substances that you have been eating that you now realize may be harmful to your liver.

_____

_____

Write a declaration about your intention to begin eating in a liver-friendly way.

_____

_____

_____

Chapter 4

Wisdom and Supplements

The Bible declares, "The wise woman builds her house, but the foolish tears it down with her own hands" (Prov. 14:1, NAS). We can conclude from this proverb that it takes wisdom to build, but foolishness tears down.

Building up your body's immune system so that it has the strength it needs to win its battle against hepatitis C requires godly wisdom. If you or a loved one has hepatitis C, strengthening your body will require making wise nutritional choices. But that is not all. Your immune system is waging a long battle and needs incredible resources to endure and overcome. That's why adding nutritional supplements can make a vital difference for you.

Supplements will provide your body with the vital resources it needs to give it strength and endurance to meet and beat the challenge it is facing. The supplements we will discuss are recommended for all stages of hepatitis C except cirrhosis of the liver. People suffering from cirrhosis must be closely monitored by their physician, and supplements may need to be reduced according to their doctor's recommendations.

Get a Really Good Multivitamin

Our bodies are unable to make sufficient quantities of most vitamins. In addition, we do not get many of these vitamins in the foods we eat because our food supply is devitalized. That's because farming methods and processing procedures often destroy much of the nutritional value of the foods we eat. By the time our food gets to the table, it has lost so much nutritional value that our bodies continue to crave what they need.

Patients with hepatitis C must avoid vitamin and mineral deficiencies since this will directly affect the immune system and may accelerate the disease process leading to fibrosis, cirrhosis of the liver and even liver cancer.

Always start your supplement program with a good comprehensive multivitamin/mineral supplement. A comprehensive multivitamin, such as our own Divine Health Multivitamin, is absolutely essential for the health of all patients with hepatitis C. A good multivitamin should contain at least 400 IU of vitamin E, 400 IU of vitamin D, 200 micrograms of selenium, all eight of the B vitamins, vitamin C and zinc.

Taking a comprehensive multivitamin and mineral supplement will help your body to get enough

> *He forgives all my sins and heals all my diseases.*
> —Psalm 103:3

vitamins, minerals and antioxidants every day. It will give your immune system most of the raw materials it requires to do its job well.

Cautions for These Supplements

A good multivitamin/mineral formula provides a foundation for your supplementation program, giving you the balance of nutrients that you need. But it is important to understand that excessive amounts of certain vitamins and minerals can actually be dangerous to your liver. You should be aware of the following cautions regarding these supplements:

Vitamin A

Too much vitamin A can damage the liver. For

that reason, I do not recommend taking over 25,000 IU of vitamin A per day.

Vitamin D

Vitamin D is another fat-soluble vitamin that may be toxic to the liver if taken in high doses. I recommend taking 400 IU of vitamin D per day, and never recommend taking over 1,000 IU per day.

Niacin

Another vitamin that is potentially toxic to the liver when taken in high doses is niacin. Fifty milligrams of niacin per day is sufficient. However, to lower cholesterol, many doctors prescribe doses of 500 milligrams of niacin two to three times per day. This can be toxic to a patient with hepatitis C. If you are taking niacin because of elevated cholesterol, be sure and have your liver functions checked after the first month and then at least every three months. Because high doses of niacin may cause inflammation of the liver, patients with hepatitis C should be monitored more closely.

Iron

If you have hepatitis C, you should not take any supplemental iron unless your doctor advises it. The hepatitis C virus actually needs iron to thrive.

That's why patients with high iron levels are more prone to experience the progression of the hepatitis C to fibrosis, cirrhosis and even liver cancer.

So, never supplement with a multivitamin tablet that contains iron, and never take supplemental iron if you have hepatitis C. This is another reason why you should dramatically decrease your consumption of red meat to only one time a week or less frequently.

Antioxidant Support

Vitamin C

High doses of vitamin C have antiviral qualities that have been known to help some individuals with hepatitis C. However, one caution when considering a higher dose of vitamin C is that it may cause increased uptake of iron from the gastrointestinal tract. In other words, it can help your body absorb even more iron from your food. We mentioned that iron promotes the disease process for hepatitis C. If you take high doses of vitamin C (over 1000 milligrams a day), be sure to have your serum iron and ferritin levels checked by your physician.

Avoid or decrease consumption of the iron-rich foods listed on page 40. You can call

(800) LEAD-OUT to find a nutritional doctor to administer vitamin C by IV.

Beyond C is an excellent high-dose vitamin C supplement that can be ordered by calling (800) 580-7587. I recommend 1 teaspoon two to three times a day. However, start with ½ teaspoon three times a day.

Alpha-lipoic acid

One of the best supplements you can take for protecting the liver is alpha-lipoic acid. This powerful antioxidant does its work of fighting and extinguishing free radicals, which cause a great deal of damage at the cellular level.

Some antioxidants are only effective in certain areas of the body where they can be absorbed, such as fat-soluble or water-soluble tissues. However, alpha-lipoic acid is powerfully effective in tissues throughout the body. In addition to that, it helps the body produce glutathione, which is another powerful antioxidant that protects liver cells and destroys viruses.

Alpha-lipoic acid is the only antioxidant that can recycle or renew itself as well as recycle other antioxidants, including vitamin E, vitamin C, coenzyme Q-10 and glutathione.[1] Let me explain. When most antioxidants donate an electron, it is used up. But alpha-lipoic acid recycles its electrons so that it can continue to perform its antioxidant functions.

These are some of the powerful effects alpha-lipoic acid has on the body:

- It helps to protect the liver.
- It aids in regenerating the liver.
- It stimulates the immune system.
- It reduces the risk of developing cirrhosis and liver cancer.

With all of these incredible benefits, it's easy to see why this supplement is considered by some to be the most important supplement for hepatitis C. Our formulated Divine Health Lipoic Acid contains 300 milligrams of alpha-lipoic acid and is pharmaceutical grade, which means it is of the highest quality.

I recommend taking 300 milligrams of alpha-lipoic acid two to three times a day.

Amino Acids Can Help

N-acetyl cysteine (NAC)

One of the most important amino acids that you can take for your liver is N-acetyl cysteine, otherwise known as NAC. NAC is hepatoprotective, which means it is a liver protector. In addition to that, it also acts as a powerful antioxidant.

Supplementing with NAC enables your body to make its own glutathione, the powerful antioxidant that protects the liver. In other words, it is a "precursor" of glutathione. Some feel the key to its special liver protection qualities is its ability to increase the levels of glutathione within liver cells.

I recommend 500 milligrams of NAC twice a day, taken with food.

SAM-e

SAM-e is an amino acid that helps to prevent a fatty liver. A fatty liver is usually associated with alcoholism, obesity or diabetes and involves fatty changes in the liver cells from fat deposits in the cells. A fatty liver also may cause inflammation of the liver.

SAM-e is useful as well in treating depression that commonly accompanies hepatitis C. If your liver does not have enough of its own SAM-e, it cannot eliminate the amino acid methionine, which can build up to toxic levels.

If you are experiencing depression and have hepatitis C, I recommend taking 200 milligrams of SAM-e (one or two tablets) twice a day on an empty stomach.

Glandular Supplements

Your thymus is a gland located in the base of your neck behind the top part of your breastbone. This powerfully important gland secretes hormones that help to regulate your immune system. These hormones include thymosin, thymopoietin and serum thymic factor.

Experts believe that thymosin can actually energize your body's immune system, helping it to fight hepatitis C. It also may help your body to produce more interferon, which is a powerful virus-fighting substance. Researchers are presently studying this powerful hormone in combination with interferon for the treatment of hepatitis C virus, and they are seeing exciting results. Thymic extract, such as NatCell frozen thymus extract, is being given to hepatitis C patients under the tongue to help bolster their immune systems.

Lloyd Wright describes his personal testimony of triumphing over hepatitis C in his book *Triumph Over Hepatitis C.*[2] In his recovery he used NatCell Thymus, along with vitamins, herbs and various nutritional therapies. He believes that his victory over hepatitis C is largely due to taking NatCell Thymus.

Wright actually took one vial of NatCell Thymus every other day for eighteen months, something that would be very expensive to do. However, it proved to be very effective for Mr. Wright, as it has been for many others who have used this supplement.[3]

Healing Herbs

In addition to these supplements that can dramatically benefit your body in its battle against hepatitis C, a number of healing herbs can make a real difference, as well. Here are some herbs that you can add to your supplement program in your battle against this disease.

Milk thistle

I personally believe the most important herb to use in the treatment of hepatitis C is milk thistle. Milk thistle contains a substance called silymarin, which blocks the formation of leukotrienes (substances in your cells involved in inflammation that damage your liver's cells). Silymarin helps your damaged liver to regenerate liver tissue, as well as protects your liver from the damaging effects of the hepatitis virus.

That's not all. This powerful substance also goes to work acting as an antioxidant and quenching free-radical damage. It also is believed to help prevent glutathione deficiency in the liver cells.

Milk thistle may well be the most powerful herb for both protecting the liver against toxins that damage it and repairing damaged liver tissue. Taking milk thistle commonly improves liver function tests, especially the ALT test.

I recommend taking 200 milligrams of milk thistle three times a day. Divine Health Milk Thistle is a protective, high-quality supplement. It can be ordered by calling (407) 331-7007.

Schizandra chinensis

Another powerful herb for your liver is a Chinese herb called Schizandra chinensis. The Chinese have used this herb for nearly two thousand years as a liver tonic.

Schizandra also works as a protector of the liver. It contains lignin compounds that can actually lower your ALT levels. This ancient Chinese herb helps your body to produce its own glutathione as well, and it helps to block the production of lipid peroxides (free radicals that damage the liver).

Chinese herbs are far less likely to cause adverse reactions when compared to drugs, but reactions may occur. For this reason, it is important to be under the care of a Chinese herbalist, known as a TCM practitioner, or an experienced nutritional doctor when taking Schizandra. This herb is typically used in combination with several other herbs.

I recommend Schizandra chinensis from Kan Herb Company, which is a very potent and bioavailable herbal elixir. I recommend 30 drops taken in the mouth and mixed with saliva and then swallowed three times a day. This must be prescribed by a nutritional doctor or TCM practitioner. Call (800) 543-5233 to find a doctor in your area.

Reishi mushrooms

The red-cap Reishi mushrooms grow on trees and are commonly found in Asia. Reishi mushrooms have been proven to help to normalize liver enzymes and to help protect the liver. They may even help a damaged liver to restore itself.

RM-10 incorporates twelve different Chinese and Japanese mushrooms and herbs, including Reishi mushrooms. This combination enhances natural killer cell activity and increases interferon-alpha levels. It also enhances the activity of other immune cells. Recommended dosage is to take nine tablets a day for four months, six tablets a day for four months and three tablets a day thereafter, with weekly one day off intervals. To order RM-10, call Longevity Plus at (800) 580-7587.

Chinese bupleurum

Chinese bupleurum is one of the best liver detoxifiers known. It works in several ways to help your liver fight hepatitis C. It attacks viruses, including different hepatitis viruses, and it helps to protect the liver. Bupleurum also helps to protect against numerous liver toxins and helps to prevent fatty degeneration of the liver.

I recommend Chinese bupleurum from Kan Herb Company, which is also an herbal elixir. I recommend 16–30 drops three times a day. This also must be prescribed by a nutritional doctor or TCM practitioner. Call (800) 543-5233 to find a doctor in your area.

Other helpful herbs

Burdock root, picrorhiza, dandelion root and aloe vera may also help patients with hepatitis C. However, prior to taking these herbs, consult a nutritional doctor and continue to have your liver enzymes checked periodically.

Start with a comprehensive multivitamin, lipoic acid, milk thistle, RM-10 and NatCell Thymus. If you can locate a nutritional doctor, begin

Schizandra chinensis and Chinese bupleurum.

Don't Take These Herbs!

Never take herbs indiscriminately. Not all herbs are good for your liver, especially if you have hepatitis C. Some herbs can be very toxic and could cause harm.

Here's a list of herbs to avoid if you have hepatitis C:

- Chaparral
- Comfrey root
- Germander
- Hops
- Kava
- Mate tea
- Mistletoe
- Skullcap
- Valerian
- Yohimbe

Caution: If you plan to take Chinese or American herbs as a part of your treatment for hepatitis C, it's very important to have your liver functions checked one month after beginning herbs and every three to four months thereafter. Discontinue use immediately of any herbs that cause an elevation in liver functions.

Finding a Therapy That Is Right for You

There are many pathways to healing hepatitis C. Nutrition, supplements, herbs, medications and prayer can all work together in concert in helping you to overcome this disease. There are also conventional medical treatments for hepatitis C. A brief discussion of these therapies may help you find the treatment that is right for you.

The standard treatment for hepatitis C offered today by conventional methods primarily relies upon the drug interferon. It is sometimes used in combination with another drug, ribavirin.

Used by itself, interferon has a track record of between 7 percent and 20 percent long-term improvement. In other words, between 7 percent and 20 percent of patients who take interferon experience a return to normalcy of their liver enzymes.

Not only is its success rate low, but taking interferon also compromises the general well-being of a patient. Side effects, including flu-like symptoms, depression, fatigue, decreased appetite and nausea, may persist for weeks, months or throughout the duration of therapy, which usually lasts from six to twelve months, though occasionally it lasts as long as eighteen months.

Though interferon alone isn't very effective, when combined with ribavirin there is a synergistic effect that makes the treatment much more powerful than when either drug is used separately. However, side effects of this combination therapy are very similar to those that accompany interferon treatment alone.

One benefit of the combined therapy is that the risk of relapse is much less. Studies have shown that combination therapy with interferon and ribavirin achieved a sustained virologic response (this means being clear of the virus for six months after treatment is finished) in 38 to 47 percent of patients when used for forty-eight weeks.

If you feel you are a good candidate for this conventional combined therapy, you should see a gastroenterologist or hepatologist first.

Conclusion

As you determine to build up your immune system and strengthen it against liver disease, never neglect to build up your inner man as well by seeking God. Determine to seek God for all of your health needs and questions. With God's help, you will be able to develop a wise strategy for healing that will be blessed with His healing touch.

The psalmist declared a wonderful testimony:

I sought the LORD, and He answered me,

and delivered me from all my fears. They looked to Him and were radiant, and their faces shall never be ashamed. This poor man cried and the LORD heard him; and saved him out of all his troubles. The angel of the LORD encamps around those who fear Him, and rescues them.

PSALM 34:4–7, NAS

Those who seek God will find wonderful answers and deliverance from trouble. Always look to God for your answers. True wisdom is found in Christ alone. The New Testament confirms this fact: "But by His doing you are in Christ Jesus, who became to us wisdom from God, and righteousness and sanctification, and redemption" (1 Cor. 1:30, NAS). In other words, Christ is God's wisdom. So look to Him for all of your needs. He will never fail you.

A BIBLE CURE PRAYER
FOR YOU

Dear Lord Jesus, I thank You that You are my wisdom, and I thank You for making Your healing wisdom available to me. Thank You for meeting all of my needs. Please help me to develop a supplement and treatment strategy that is genuinely blessed with Your wonderful wisdom and, more importantly, with Your healing power. Like the psalmist, I'm crying out to You for all of my needs. Rescue my life and save me—body, soul and spirit. Thank You that it's accomplished already! In Jesus' name, amen.

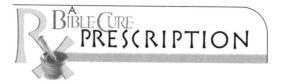

Check supplements that you intend to consult your medical provider about taking.

- ❏ A comprehensive multivitamin, such as Divine Health Multivitamin, that contains vitamin E, vitamin D, 200 mcg. of selenium, vitamin C, zinc and all eight B vitamins
- ❏ Alpha-lipoic acid
- ❏ NAC
- ❏ NatCell Thymus
- ❏ Milk thistle
- ❏ Schizandra chinensis
- ❏ Reishi mushrooms (RM-10)
- ❏ Chinese bupleurum

Look up James 1:5 and write a few sentences about how you will apply this scripture to your situation.

_____

_____

_____

Chapter 5

Wisdom and Healing Through Prayer

God's wisdom for hepatitis and hepatitis C includes powerful spiritual tools, including prayer for healing:

> Are any among you sick? They should call for the elders of the church and have them pray over them, anointing them with oil in the name of the Lord. And their prayer offered in faith will heal the sick, and the Lord will make them well. And anyone who has committed sins will be forgiven.
>
> —JAMES 5:14–15

If you are fighting hepatitis or hepatitis C, a vital part of God's Bible cure for you is prayer. Ask your pastor and other friends who believe in prayer to lay hands on you and anoint you with oil for healing. You have God's promise that prayer can make all the difference in the world. The Bible declares, "The earnest prayer of a righteous person has great power and wonderful results" (James 5:16).

Medical Science Confirms
Benefits of Prayer

Even the medical community is beginning to take notice of the wonderful benefits of healing prayer. As a matter of fact, the powerful results of prayer for healing are being studied scientifically with amazing results. Researchers Mitchell Krucoff and Suzanne Crater conducted a study on how prayer by strangers affected the outcome of cardiovascular patients at Duke University Hospital in Durham, North Carolina. Early results of the study showed that the outcomes of those receiving prayer were 50 to 100 percent better than a control group that received no prayer.[1]

Another study, published in the *Journal of the American Medical Association* (*JAMA*) by Randolph Byrd of the San Francisco Medical Center, discovered that patients who were prayed over suffered far few complications following surgery. And in 1995, a study done at Darmouth-

Hitchcock Medical Center found that one of the best predictors of survival among 232 heart-surgery patients was the degree to which the patients said they drew comfort and strength from religious faith. Those who did not confess religious faith had more than three times the death rate of those who did.[2]

God's Promise of Healing

God's promises of healing are very real—enough to be medically documented by those who do not even believe in God! This should encourage you to make the choice to believe in God for healing. He desires for you to be well because He loves you very deeply, with a greater love than you can even comprehend.

God's Word declares His great love for you and the many benefits He provides for His children:

> Bless the Lord, O my soul,
> And forget none of His benefits;
> Who pardons all your iniquities;
> Who heals all your diseases;
> Who redeems your life from the pit;
> Who crowns you with loving-kindness and
> compassion;
> Who satisfies your years with good things,

So that your youth is renewed like the
eagle.

—Psalm 103:2–5, nas

God's love for you is deeper than the ocean and
higher than the sky. It's not God's will for you to
die an early death; it's His will for you to live a life
of health and wholeness. The apostle Paul prayed
that we might know the height and the depth of
the love that is in Christ Jesus. (See Ephesians
3:18–19.) That's my prayer for you today, too,
that you might know God's great expansive love
and experience His loving, healing touch upon
your body right now.

Faith for Healing

Jesus Christ taught that any mountain of sickness
and disease will move when faith is applied. He
said, "I assure you, even if you had faith as small
as a mustard seed you could say to this mountain,
'Move from here to there,' and it would move.
Nothing would be impossible" (Matt. 17:20).

Let me teach you a powerful secret about faith.
Faith is the greatest force in the whole universe.
Absolutely nothing is impossible to a person with
faith. But listen carefully. Faith is not a feeling or
an emotion. It is not a cloud or a dove or a power

that comes upon certain people. Faith is a choice—pure and simple. Faith is a decision to believe God's promise despite circumstances and feelings that seem to be contrary.

I have watched faith move many mountains. I have seen many people rise from wheelchairs and be healed by the power of the Holy Spirit. Those individuals are not different from you. They had no less doubt or discouragement. They didn't think higher thoughts or come from more godly families. They simply chose to believe God. Faith is so simple!

A Faith Prescription

Here's a faith prescription that I want you to take just as faithfully as you would a medicine. Confess aloud by faith the following at least three times per day: *I believe that by Your stripes, Lord Jesus, I am healed of hepatitis C.*

Healing for Dangerous Emotions

Many years ago, Hans Selye, in his book *The Stress of Life*, demonstrated that prolonged stress could wear down certain vital organs in the body.[3] For example, you have probably heard of the adrenal glands in relation to the stress hormone adrenaline. Stress affects a part of the adrenal gland, called the adrenal cortex, so negatively that it causes it to become enlarged. Stress also wears away the thymus, spleen and lymph nodes, and can cause bleeding ulcers.

Selye showed that unrelieved stress leads to elevation of the hormone *cortisol* in the blood. A number of deadly conditions are linked to high cortisol levels, including hypertension, ulcers, depression, cancer, diabetes, arthritis, stroke, heart disease, alcoholism and drug addiction.

Cortisol is also an immunosuppressant, which means that it suppresses the function of the immune system so needed to fight disease. High levels of cortisol in the body caused by prolonged stress can actually destroy lymphatic tissue and can damage the thymus gland, which is vitally important in helping your body overcome hepatitis C. Increased levels of cortisol due to stress also decrease the number of T-helper cells that help to eliminate the hepatitis C virus. You can see from this one altered hormone how devastating negative emotions can be to the health of the body.

In order to experience God's healing touch in your body, it will be necessary to deal with the negative emotions that can be a part of liver disease. As we mentioned earlier, Chinese doctors have believed for centuries that the liver is the seat of negative emotions. In other words, dark emotions such as anger, frustration and rage stress the liver, leading to disease.

Choosing a lifestyle of prayer and declaring the Word of God, as well as dwelling in an atmosphere of praise and worship, can all work together to strengthen your immune system, resulting in delay and even prevention of the progression of hepatitis C to cirrhosis and liver cancer. Combined with your faith, these spiritual weapons can work powerfully in helping you receive your healing.

A scientific study published in *JAMA* by Randolph Byrd of the San Francisco Medical Center found that the laying on of hands in prayer relieves stress better than drugs.[4]

In addition, other negative emotions linked to liver disease are also much less involved among hepatitis C patients who practice a life of faith. A 1996 National Institute study on aging of four thousand elderly living at home in North Carolina found that those who attend religious services are less depressed and physically healthier than those who don't attend or who worship at home.[5]

In another study of thirty elderly female patients recovering from hip fractures, those who regarded God as a source of strength and comfort and who attended religious services were able to walk farther upon discharge and had lower rates of depression than those who expressed no faith in God.[6]

God does not intend for us to go it alone. Don't try to deal with your hepatitis C by yourself. Surround yourself with others who have faith for your healing, and become a worshiper yourself. Singing and worshiping God can release a sense of joy and peace

> *The Spirit of the Lord is upon me, for he has appointed me to preach Good News to the poor. He has sent me to proclaim that captives will be released, that the blind will see, that the downtrodden will be freed from their oppressors.*
> —Luke 4:18

into your body and mind that has a wonderfully healing effect.

Join a prayer group or a Sunday school class that will help you to keep your mind focused on the Word of God. God's Word is very powerful. The scriptures declare, "He sent His word and healed them, and delivered them from their destructions" (Ps. 107:20, NAS).

A Prescription for Laughter

How long has it been since you've had a good belly laugh—you know, the kind that brings tears to your eyes and changes the way you feel for the rest of the day? According to God's Word, laughter has as much healing power as medicine. In Proverbs we read, "A cheerful heart is good medicine" (Prov. 17:22).

A good belly laugh actually massages your internal organs. It releases tension, anxiety, anger, fear, shame and guilt, and it transforms your attitude and outlook on life.

So, here's another healing prescription: Laugh until it hurts. Pick up a good comedy video or a funny joke book and let yourself laugh. Laugh heartily and often. Take a laughter break three times per day.

Find a Support Group

I advise all my patients who have hepatitis C to join a support group. Support group members are more likely to get breaking news on new medications, vitamins, herbs or other treatments for hepatitis C as they become available. Members of the support group also understand the disease, symptoms and frustrations you experience on a day-to-day basis, and they are able to offer a sympathetic ear to your concerns. Patients who are part of a support group are better able to cope with their disease, treatment and even side effects of treatments as well as negative emotional responses.

It is critically important to find a knowledgeable doctor who has treated hundreds of patients with hepatitis C. Most family practitioners are inexperienced in treating hepatitis C. Therefore, I recommend that you see either a gastroenterologist or hepatologist. When you are a member of a good support group, you will have the opportunity to find doctors experienced in treating hepatitis C. That's the best way to find a good doctor.

I also strongly recommend that you find a good nutritional doctor or a Chinese herbalist who can assist you in making good choices. Hopefully this small booklet will be a helpful nutritional guide in the meantime. Remember, the hepatitis C virus thrives on alcohol, drugs, medications, sugar, iron, junk foods, anger, frustration, depression and a defeated attitude. When added to faith, good nutrition and a positive attitude will go a long ways to get you into the healing process. (For more information on the effects of stress, please refer to my booklet *The Bible Cure for Stress*.)

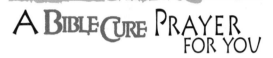

A BIBLE CURE PRAYER
FOR YOU

Dear Lord, help me to make all the wisdom I've received throughout this Bible cure a living reality in my life. Thank You for Your great love and healing power. Reveal that expansive love to me in an entirely new and thrilling way. I choose to trust You for my health and healing, and I thank You that You will never fail me. Right now I declare that I believe in Your love, and I commit my life anew to a joyous walk in Your wonderful presence. In Jesus' name, amen.

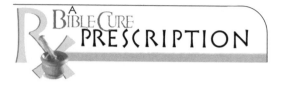

A BIBLE CURE PRESCRIPTION

What spiritual tools do you plan to use as you believe for your healing? (circle)

Worship
Personal prayer
Receiving prayer and anointing with oil for
    healing from believers
Joining a prayer group
Joining a Bible study group
Attending church
Thanking God for healing
Reading God's Word
Practicing joy and laughter
Confessing the Word of God and refusing
    to voice your fears

Write a prayer thanking God for healing you.

_____

_____

_____

A Personal Note

From Don and Mary Colbert

God desires to heal you of disease. His Word is full of promises that confirm His love for you and His desire to give you His abundant life. His desire includes more than physical health for you; He wants to make you whole in your mind and spirit as well through a personal relationship with His Son, Jesus Christ.

If you haven't met my best friend, Jesus, I would like to take this opportunity to introduce Him to you. It is very simple.

If you are ready to let Him come into your heart and become your best friend, just bow your head and sincerely pray this prayer from your heart:

> *Lord Jesus, I want to know You as my Savior and Lord. I believe You are the Son of God and that You died for my sins. I also believe You were raised from the dead and now sit at the right hand of the Father praying for me. I ask You to forgive me for my sins and change my heart so that I can*

be Your child and live with You eternally.
Thank You for Your peace. Help me to
walk with You so that I can begin to know
You as my best friend and my Lord. Amen.

If you have prayed this prayer, we rejoice with you in your decision and your new relationship with Jesus. Please contact us at pray4me@strang.com so that we can send you some materials that will help you become established in your relationship with the Lord. You have just made the most important decision of your life. We look forward to hearing from you.

Notes

CHAPTER 3: WISDOM AND NUTRITION

1. Roberta Duyff, *The American Dietetic Association's Complete Food and Nutrition Guide* (Minneapolis, MN: Chronimed Publishing, 1998).

CHAPTER 4: WISDOM AND SUPPLEMENTS

1. Lester Packer, *The Antioxidant Miracle* (New York: John Wiley and Sons, Inc., 1999).
2. Lloyd Wright, *Triumph Over Hepatitis C* (Malibu, CA: Lloyd Wright Publishing, 2000).
3. You can get more information about this powerful supplement from Lloyd Wright's own website at www.hepatitiscfree.com.

CHAPTER 5: WISDOM AND HEALING THROUGH PRAYER

1. David Van Biema, "A Test of the Healing Power of Prayer," *Time* (October 12, 1998).
2. Claudia Wallis, "Faith and Healing," *Time* (June 24, 1996).
3. Hans Selye, *The Stress of Life* (New York: McGraw-Hill, 1978).
4. Wallis, "Faith and Healing."
5. Ibid.
6. Ibid.

Don Colbert, M.D., was born in Tupelo, Mississippi. He attended Oral Roberts School of Medicine in Tulsa, Oklahoma, where he received a bachelor of science degree in biology in addition to his degree in medicine. Dr. Colbert completed his internship and residency with Florida Hospital in Orlando, Florida. He is board certified in family practice and has received extensive training in nutritional medicine.

If you would like more
information about natural and
divine healing, or information about
Divine Health Nutritional Products®,
you may contact
Dr. Colbert at:

DR. DON COLBERT

1908 Boothe Circle
Longwood, FL 32750
Telephone: 407-331-7007
(For ordering products only)

Dr. Colbert's website is
www.drcolbert.com.

Disclaimer: Dr. Colbert and the staff of Divine Health Wellness Center are prohibited from addressing a patient's medical condition by phone, facsimile or e-mail. Please refer questions related to your medical condition to your own primary care physician.